HEADACHE-FREE LIVING

Mind-Body Methods, Dietary Strategies, And Trigger Identification For Headache Management

Dr. ATHENA ABELL

Table of Contents

CHAPTER ONE

Introduction

Headaches are a prevalent medical condition that affects a significant number of people at different stages throughout their lifetimes. Headaches, which may be caused by tension, stress, or other variables, have the potential to greatly disrupt daily activities and overall health.

Gaining a comprehensive understanding of the complex interplay between the mind and body is essential for devising efficacious strategies to prevent and manage migraines. This investigation examines the correlation between migraines and the mind-body dynamic, providing perspectives on strategies for mitigating and averting headaches through dietary modifications, stress reduction techniques, relaxation methods, and yoga.

Comprehension Of Headaches

A variety of headache types can present themselves, such as tension headaches, migraines, and cluster headaches, each possessing distinct attributes. Migraines are distinguished by intense pulsating pain, vertigo, and extreme sensitivity to light and sound, whereas tension headaches are frequently brought on by muscle tension or stress. Cluster migraines, while infrequent, are severe and frequently manifest in succession over a specific time frame.

Headaches can be induced by a multitude of factors, including physical, psychological, and environmental influences. Determining the precise etiology of an individual's migraines is an essential component in the formulation of efficacious management approaches.

The interrelation between the psyche and body is substantial, and this correlation influences the development and treatment of migraines.

Anxiety, stress, and emotional tension are all psychological elements that may contribute to the onset and worsening of migraines. Physical factors such as muscle tension, posture, and dehydration may also contribute.

Gaining comprehension of the mind-body connection empowers individuals to embrace holistic methodologies that attend to the physical and mental dimensions. Through stress management, the implementation of relaxation techniques, and the promotion of holistic well-being, it is feasible to mitigate the occurrence and severity of migraines.

Stress Mitigation Methods

migraines are frequently induced by tension; therefore, integrating stress reduction strategies into one's daily routine can serve as a crucial measure in both mitigating and averting migraines. Effective techniques for reducing tension include:

1. Deep breathing exercises have the potential to induce the body's relaxation response, thereby aiding in the alleviation of stress and tension. Practicing guided breathing exercises and diaphragmatic breathing can be effortlessly integrated into one's daily regimen.

2. Progressive Muscle Relaxation (PMR): In PMR, various muscle groups in the body are systematically contracted and then relaxed. By aiding in the release of bodily tension and fostering general relaxation, this practice is advantageous in the prevention of headaches.

3. The practice of mindfulness entails directing one's attention to the current instant without passing judgment on it. By increasing an individual's awareness of their thoughts and sensations, mindful meditation can alleviate the physical and mental effects of stress.

CHAPTER TWO

Meditation And Relaxation

Methods of relaxation and meditation are effective strategies for the management of headaches. Consistent practice has the potential to improve one's overall state of being and foster a feeling of tranquility.

By integrating techniques such as progressive muscle relaxation, mindfulness meditation, and guided imagery into one's daily regimen, it is possible to cultivate a state of tranquility that encompasses both the body and mind, thereby diminishing the probability of experiencing migraines.

Yoga To Alleviate Headaches

Yoga is a comprehensive discipline comprising meditation, physical postures, and respiration regulation. Specific yoga poses and sequences, when utilized as a supplementary strategy to headache management, have the potential to alleviate discomfort and avert the recurrence of migraines. Yoga enhances overall body awareness, improves posture, and promotes flexibility.

Yoga poses that potentially offer respite from headaches include the following:

1. Child's Pose (Balasana) is a restorative posture that assists in the alleviation of tension in the shoulders and neck, regions that are frequently linked to tension migraines.

2. Forward Fold (Uttanasana): By promoting relaxation and relieving tension in the back and neck, forward folds may alleviate the symptoms of headaches.

3. Cat-Cow Stretch (Marjaryasana-Bitilasana): This fluid transition between two postures can alleviate

tension in the back and neck and increase spinal flexibility.

4. Legs Up the Wall Pose (Viparita Karani): By increasing blood circulation, this restorative inversion aids in headache relief and promotes relaxation.

Dietary Factors To Consider

The management of headaches is influenced by dietary factors, and making informed decisions regarding food and beverages can positively impact one's overall health. Take into account the subsequent dietary considerations:

1. Inconsistent meal timing may be a contributing factor to the development of migraines. Balanced and consistent diets are essential for stabilizing blood sugar levels.

2. Identify Trigger Foods: Caffeine, chocolate, and artificial sweeteners are examples of substances and additives that may induce migraines in some people. Specific triggers can be identified and avoided with the aid of a food journal.

3. Dehydration is a frequent contributor to the development of migraines. Consistent water

consumption promotes overall health and aids in the prevention of migraines.

Headaches And Hydration

Hydration is an essential factor in the prevention of headaches. Alterations in electrolyte balance and blood volume can result from dehydration, which may induce cephalalgia. To ensure adequate hydration:

1. It is recommended to consume a minimum of eight glasses of water daily, with adjustments made according to individual

requirements, climate conditions, and level of physical activity.

2. Caffeine and alcohol should be consumed in moderation, as they can both contribute to dehydration when consumed in excess. It is essential to maintain a balance and exercise moderation.

3. Incorporate Hydrating Foods: Incorporate water-rich foods, such as fruits and vegetables, into your diet. Additionally, broths and soups can aid in hydration.

In summary, migraines are intricate occurrences comprising physical and psychological elements. Comprehending the interrelation between the mind and body, implementing relaxation techniques, engaging in yoga, selecting well-informed dietary options, and prioritizing adequate hydration are all fundamental components of a comprehensive strategy for the management and prevention of migraines.

By attending to a range of factors that contribute to migraines, individuals have the potential to improve their overall state of being and mitigate the disruptions that these distressing experiences cause in their daily routines.

CHAPTER THREE

An Examination And Treatment Of Headaches From A Holistic Perspective

Headaches, although prevalent, can have a substantial effect on one's daily functioning, productivity, and general state of being.

Although medication may offer some degree of respite from migraines, a comprehensive approach that considers multiple contributing factors can be highly effective in mitigating their incidence. This all-encompassing approach involves the identification of dietary triggers, the optimization of nutrition, the integration of regular exercise, the maintenance of good sleep hygiene, the recognition of hormonal influences, and the awareness of environmental factors.

Recognition Of Food Triggers

A critical component of headache management entails the identification and effective management of potential food triggers. Specific food items and beverages have the potential to induce migraines in those who are susceptible. Caffeine, alcoholic beverages, chocolate, aged cheese, and processed foods that contain additives such as monosodium glutamate are typical offenders. Individuals who maintain a detailed food diary may be able to identify correlations between their diet and headache episodes, thereby empowering them to make more informed decisions regarding their dietary consumption.

Dietary modifications and an awareness of personal sensitivities are effective methods for substantially mitigating the frequency and severity of migraines. Notably, individual triggers can differ; therefore, effective headache management requires a personalized approach to identifying and eliminating specific foods.

Nutrition For The Prevention Of Headaches

In addition to having a significant impact on overall health, nutrition can also affect the frequency and intensity of headaches. The fact that migraines are frequently induced by dehydration underscores the significance of maintaining proper hydration levels throughout the day. A balanced diet consisting primarily of lean proteins, fruits, vegetables, and whole cereals is crucial for obtaining vital nutrients that support overall health and potentially aid in the prevention of migraines.

Consistent and well-balanced meals can also aid in the maintenance of stable blood sugar levels, thereby mitigating the risk of headache-inducing fluctuations. By limiting their intake of processed foods, saccharine munchies, and artificial sweeteners, individuals can enhance their ability to regulate their blood sugar and decrease their susceptibility to migraines.

Fitness And Physical Exertion

Engaging in consistent physical activity is not solely advantageous for one's general well-being; it may also contribute to the prevention of migraines. Engaging in physical activity yields several positive effects, including tension reduction, mood enhancement, and improved circulation, all of which are potential preventive measures against headaches.

Participating in physical activities such as vigorous walking, jogging, cycling, or yoga is efficacious in the management of stress and tension, both of which are prevalent factors contributing to migraines.

It is critical to select activities that correspond with personal preferences and levels of physical fitness to maintain a consistent exercise regimen.

CHAPTER FOUR

Bedtime Hygiene

Sleep deprivation can contribute to the development of migraines, whereas sufficient and high-quality sleep is vital for overall hygiene. It is critical to develop and adhere to sound sleep hygiene practices to mitigate the risk of sleep-related migraines.

Creating an environment that is conducive to sleep by maintaining a calm, dark, and silent bedroom can facilitate restful slumber. Improving sleep quality can be achieved by adhering to a regular sleep regimen and avoiding stimulants such as caffeine in the hours leading up to bedtime. Additionally, the implementation of relaxation techniques, such as deep breathing or meditation, and the reduction of screen time before nighttime can contribute to improved sleep quality.

The Impact Of Hormones On Headaches

Particularly in women, hormonal fluctuations may significantly contribute to the development of migraines. A considerable number of women encounter headaches or menstrual migraines that are linked to hormonal fluctuations that occur throughout the menstrual cycle.

It is imperative to comprehend the impacts of hormones and collaborate with healthcare practitioners to devise effective approaches for regulating hormonal fluctuations. Hormonal contraception might be a feasible alternative for certain individuals, whereas others might discover alleviation via lifestyle modifications or specialized medications designed to target the causes of hormonal headaches.

Both internal and external environmental factors have the potential to induce migraines. External factors may encompass elements such as weather fluctuations, and exposure to pungent aromas, or pollutants. Internal factors consist of emotional health and tension levels.

To identify and manage environmental triggers, one must be aware of their surroundings and, whenever possible, make adjustments. Potential measures to mitigate stress include restricting the presence of pungent odors, ensuring adequate ventilation, and incorporating relaxation or mindfulness exercises as stress-reduction strategies.

In conclusion, for effective prevention, it is crucial to adopt a holistic approach to identifying and managing the various factors that contribute to migraines. Through the identification of food triggers, the optimization of nutrition, the integration of regular exercise, the maintenance of good sleep hygiene, the recognition of hormonal influences, and the awareness of environmental factors, individuals can adopt a proactive stance to mitigate the daily burden of migraines. This all-encompassing approach enables individuals to make knowledgeable decisions regarding their lifestyles, which in turn enhance their general health and reduce the occurrence and severity of migraines.

Technology And The Management Of Screen Time

Screens have become an integral part of contemporary existence, permeating nearly all facets of our daily lives. Although this connectivity facilitates communication and productivity, overindulgence in screen time may lead to adverse effects on both physical and mental well-being. Extended periods of screen time, whether originating from electronic devices such as computers, smartphones, or similar devices, have been linked to symptoms including eye strain, disruptions in sleep patterns, and migraines.

Setting boundaries, taking pauses, and adhering to the 20-20-20 rule are all components of screen time management. This rule stipulates that every 20 minutes, one should gaze at an object located 20 feet away for a minimum of 20 seconds.

Identification And Treatment Of Tension Headaches

Tension migraines, which are frequently associated with muscle tension and stress, are a prevalent condition in the fast-paced society of today. A diffuse, persistent discomfort typically manifests in the region encompassing the head, neck, and shoulders. Techniques for reducing stress, including meditation, deep breathing exercises, and regular physical activity, are utilized to manage tension migraines. In addition, proper ergonomics, a consistent sleep schedule, and adequate hydration can aid in the relief of tension migraines.

CHAPTER FIVE

Migraines are classified as neurological disorders that manifest as intense cephalalgias, frequently accompanied by symptoms such as vertigo, light and sound sensitivity, and visual impairments.

Migraine identification and treatment necessitate a comprehensive strategy. Migraine-prone people should maintain a journal to record triggers and patterns, thereby facilitating improved prevention. Lifestyle adjustments, such as adhering to a consistent sleep schedule, maintaining adequate hydration, and consuming a well-balanced diet, are critical components in the management of migraines. Furthermore, the integration of stress management and relaxation techniques into a comprehensive strategy for alleviating the frequency and severity of migraines is imperative.

Causes of Cluster Headaches and Coping Mechanisms

Cluster headaches, while less frequent than tension headaches and migraines, manifest in cyclical

In Regarding Migraines

patterns and are characterized by excruciating pain. Comprehending the etiology of cluster migraines is vital to develop efficacious managed approaches. Alcohol consumption, smoking, and specific environmental factors may serve as triggers.

Adjustments to one's lifestyle, including the avoidance of known triggers and the prompt pursuit of medical attention in the event of an episode, constitute coping mechanisms. Assistance from healthcare professionals can offer customized approaches to effectively managing the distinct difficulties presented by cluster migraines.

Medication Administration

A substantial number of patients who suffer from severe or chronic migraines incorporate medication management as an essential component of their treatment regimen.

Prescription medications, over-the-counter analgesics, and preventative drugs are frequently suggested by the nature and intensity of migraines. Strict collaboration with healthcare professionals is imperative to determine the optimal medication regimen. Consistent and ongoing communication with a healthcare provider is essential for monitoring the efficacy of medications and identifying any potential adverse effects. This promotes a proactive and personalized approach to managing headaches.

Non-Conventional Therapies

In recent times, alternative therapies for the management of headaches have garnered increasing attention, especially from those in search of holistic and complementary methodologies. These therapeutic modalities comprise an extensive range, incorporating biofeedback, aromatherapy, and herbal remedies. The integration of alternative therapies into a holistic approach to headache management necessitates meticulous deliberation of personal inclinations and requirements. When considering personal health objectives that are consistent with evidence-based and risk-free alternative therapies, it is recommended to seek guidance from healthcare professionals.

Acupuncture For The Relief Of Headaches

Ancestral acupuncture, which originated in ancient China, has garnered attention as a possible therapeutic intervention for headaches, such as migraines. By inserting thin needles into specific locations on the body, this alternative therapy promotes energy circulation and equilibrium.

Acupuncturists may be able to reduce the frequency and severity of migraines through the use of acupuncture, providing a nonpharmacological alternative for those seeking alternatives to conventional treatments. It is imperative to consult healthcare providers before implementing any alternative therapy to guarantee its safety and appropriateness for specific cases.

Thus, a comprehensive and personalized strategy is necessary for the successful management of technology-induced screen time and diverse forms of migraines. By integrating lifestyle adjustments, stress management methodologies, and medication as needed, and investigating alternative therapeutic approaches, one can develop a holistic approach to alleviating headaches.

By acquiring knowledge about the intricacies of each variety of headache and adopting a comprehensive strategy for its management, people can improve their general state of being and reestablish authority over their day-to-day activities.

CHAPTER SIX

Chiropractic Treatment

For Discourages

Chiropractic treatment has gained significant traction among individuals in search of an alternative remedy for persistent migraines.

Chiropractors employ a non-invasive technique that centers on the alignment of the vertebrae, endeavoring to rectify any misalignments that could potentially be the cause of migraines. Through the implementation of precise adjustment techniques and spinal manipulation, chiropractors aim to optimize the functionality of the nervous system, which may result in a reduction in the frequency and intensity of headaches.

Neurofeedback And Biofeedback Are

Biofeedback and neurofeedback are novel methodologies that capitalize on the interplay between the mind and body to address headaches.

Monitoring physiological functions such as skin temperature, heart rate, and muscle tension constitutes biofeedback. By developing this consciousness, people can regulate these bodily functions, which may result in the acquisition of control over the stimuli that cause headaches.

Neurofeedback enhances this concept by emphasizing brainwave activity, to modify brain function to reduce the frequency of headaches.

Supplements And Herbal Remedies

Herbal supplements and remedies have their origins in traditional medicine practices, which date back centuries. Regarding the management of headaches, specific botanicals and supplements have garnered considerable interest due to their purported advantages. Several substances, including butterbur, feverfew, magnesium, and riboflavin, are thought to be involved in the alleviation of headaches.

It is essential, nevertheless, to exercise prudence when utilizing these remedies and to consult a professional for advice on safety and effectiveness.

Integrating Therapies to Provide
Immense Relief

Although individual alternative therapies may provide some degree of alleviation, the integration of multiple approaches frequently yields a more comprehensive and synergistic outcome.

By combining biofeedback and chiropractic care, or by integrating herbal remedies with neurofeedback, a customized approach can be developed to address multiple facets of headache triggers and symptoms. This comprehensive approach recognizes the distinctiveness of every person's headache experience and endeavors to develop an individualized resolution.

Maintaining A Headache Diary

Consisting of a headache journal is an invaluable practice for the identification of patterns and triggers. The act of documenting headache-related information such as their onset time, severity, and possible triggers enables both patients and medical professionals to identify patterns that might otherwise elude detection.

Developing this self-awareness facilitates the customization of headache management strategies.

Seeking Expert Assistance

When investigating alternative treatments for headaches, it is vital to seek the advice of medical professionals who specialize in headache management.

The expertise of chiropractors, neurofeedback specialists, and herbalists can furnish invaluable counsel and insight.

CHAPTER SEVEN

Strategies For Preventing Headaches

Prevention is frequently crucial in the management of chronic migraines. By implementing lifestyle adjustments, mastering stress management strategies, and recognizing and evading particular triggers, the frequency and intensity of migraines can be substantially diminished. The establishment of a regular sleep routine, adequate hydration, and the application of relaxation techniques are fundamental components in the prevention of migraines.

Resources And Support Systems In The Community

Experiencing chronic migraines can present significant emotional and mental challenges. Emotional strain can be mitigated through the utilization of community resources and the formation of a support network. Support groups, whether conducted virtually or in person, offer avenues for members to exchange personal anecdotes, coping mechanisms, and emotional encouragement. The presence of this communal spirit can serve as an essential element when dealing with the intricacies of managing chronic headaches.

Formulating an individualized strategy for managing headaches

As individuals examine diverse alternatives and incorporate various therapeutic approaches, their overarching objective is to formulate an individualized strategy for managing headaches. By integrating successful tactics discovered via empirical investigation, expert advice, and introspection, this strategy transforms into a versatile instrument in the continuous pursuit of alleviation from headaches.

Conclusion

When considering the management of headaches, adopting a holistic and alternative approach presents a wide range of potential outcomes that extend beyond conventional medical interventions.

An extensive array of techniques, including biofeedback, herbal remedies, chiropractic care, and biofeedback, enable individuals to customize their headache management according to their specific requirements. By integrating multiple therapeutic interventions, cultivating self-awareness via the use of a headache journal, seeking expert advice, and establishing a strong support network, individuals can develop an individualized and all-encompassing strategy for effectively managing chronic headaches. This will not only improve their overall health but also restore a feeling of agency and personal agency.